When You Feel Better

A get well soon gift for:

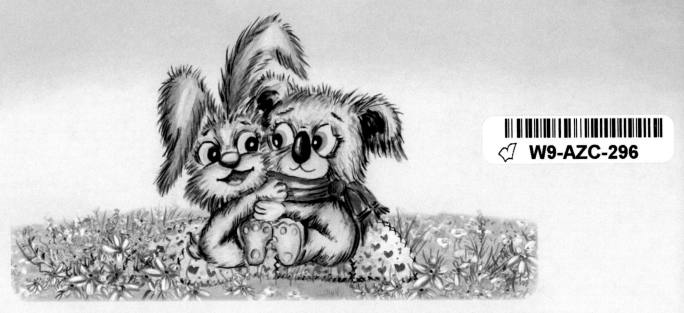

Written by **MISTY BLACK**   Artwork by **MARINA BATRAK**

Berry Patch Press LLC

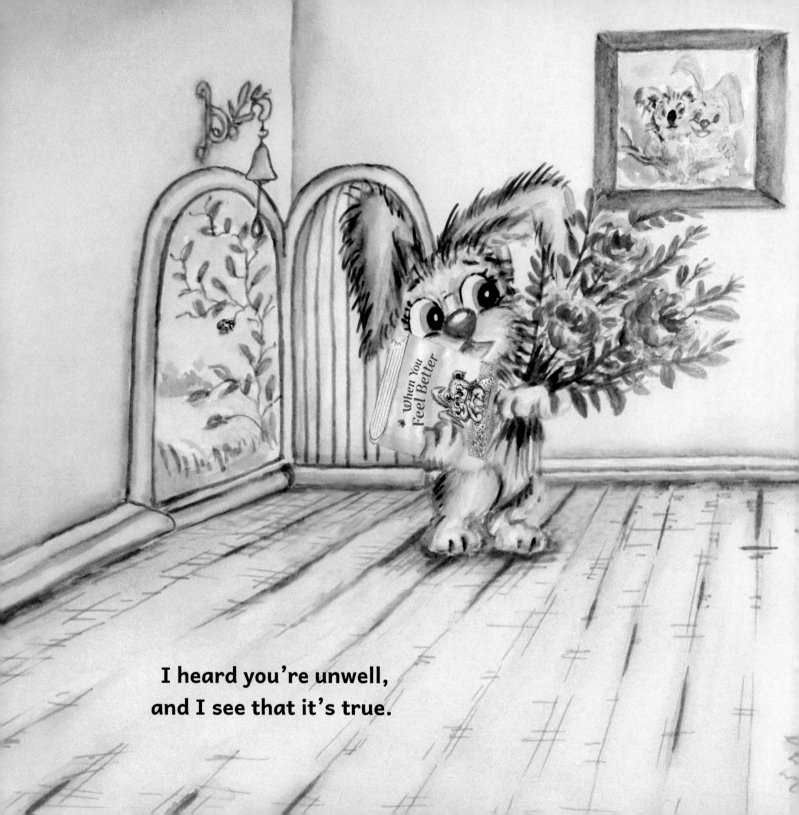

I heard you're unwell,
and I see that it's true.

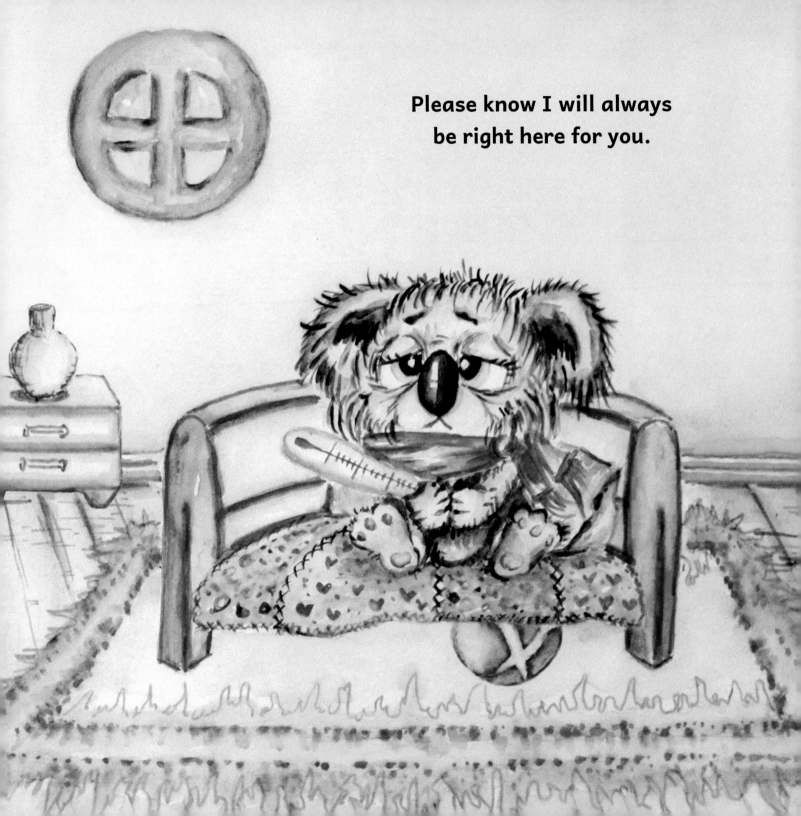

Please know I will always be right here for you.

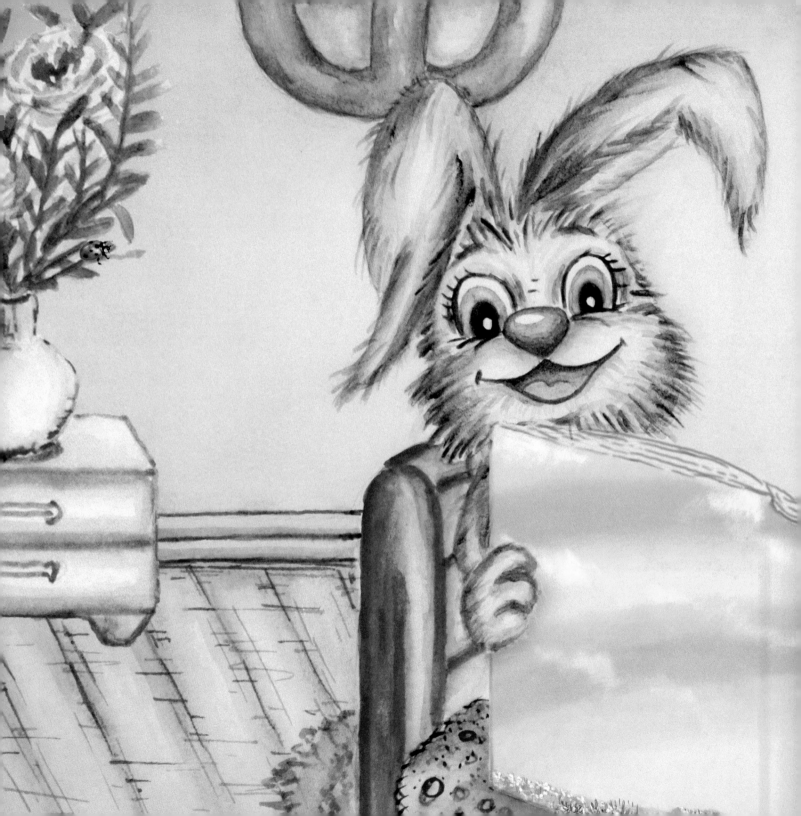

I made you this book to show you I care.
Imagine the many adventures we'll share.

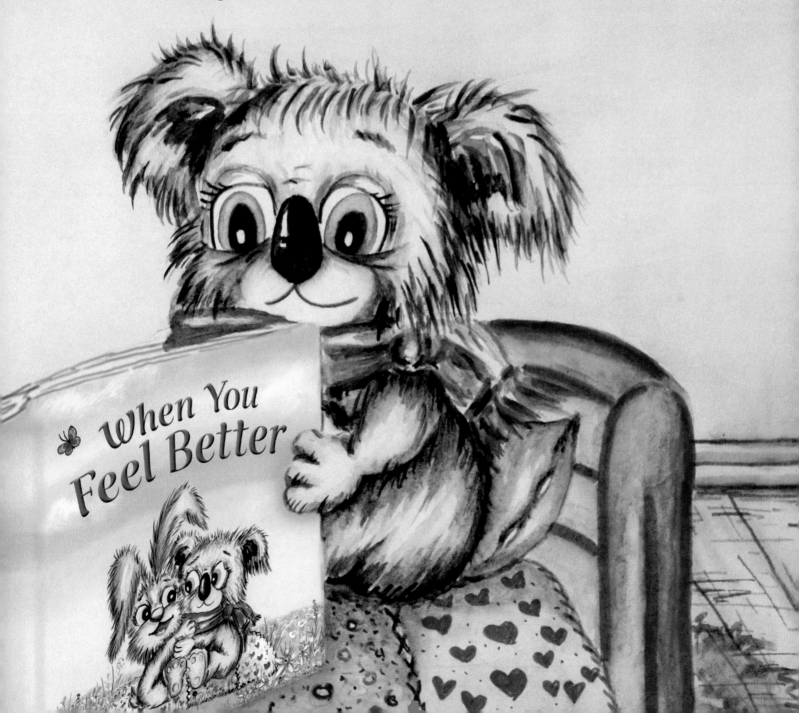

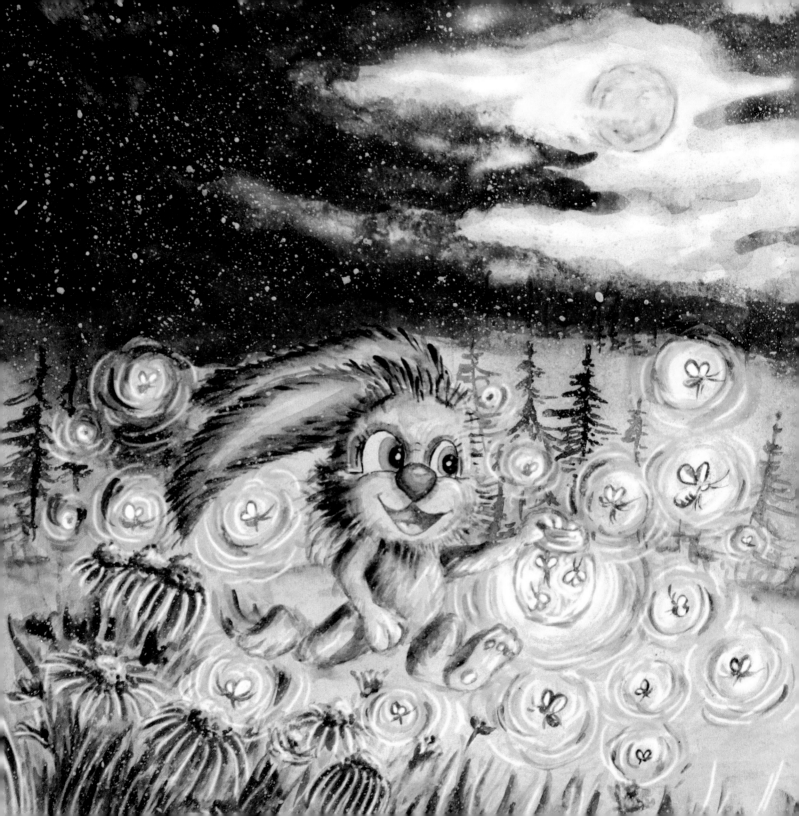

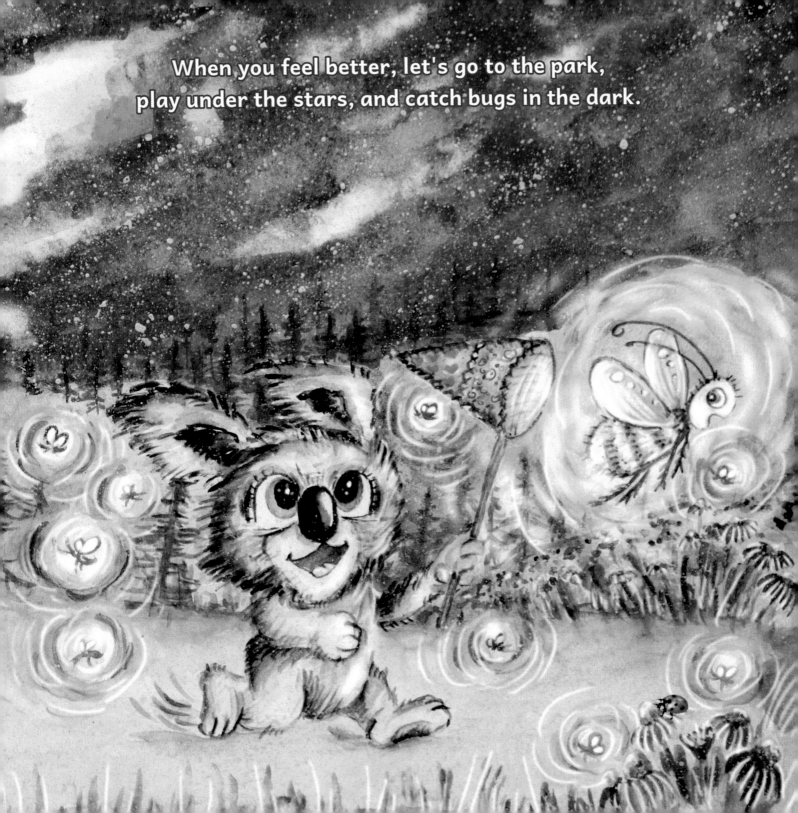

When you feel better, let's go to the park,
play under the stars, and catch bugs in the dark.

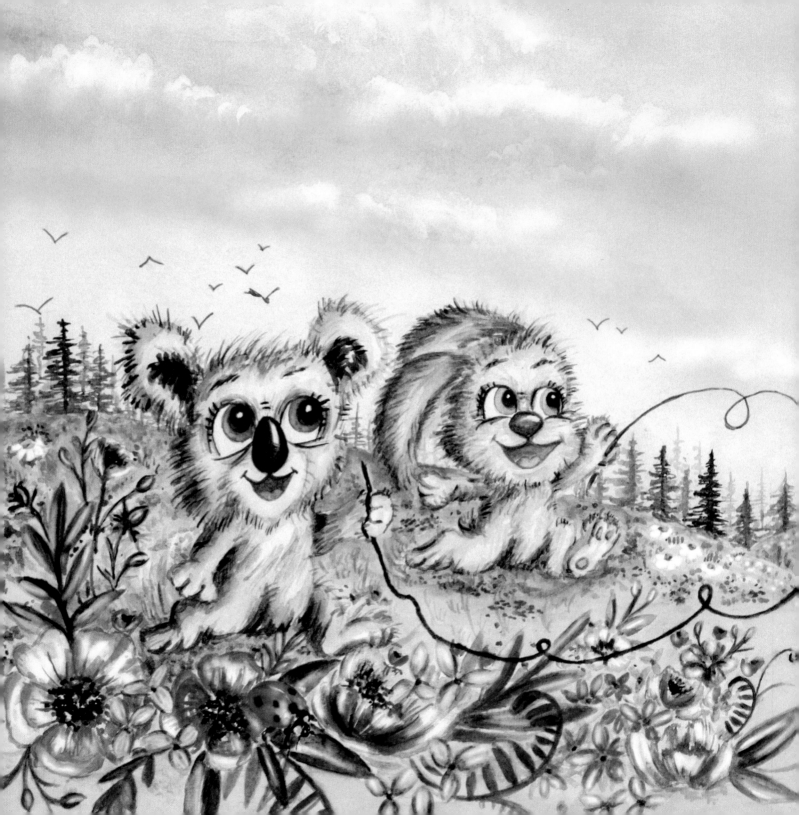

Then in the morning, we'll go for a run.
We'll fly our kites high in the warm summer sun.

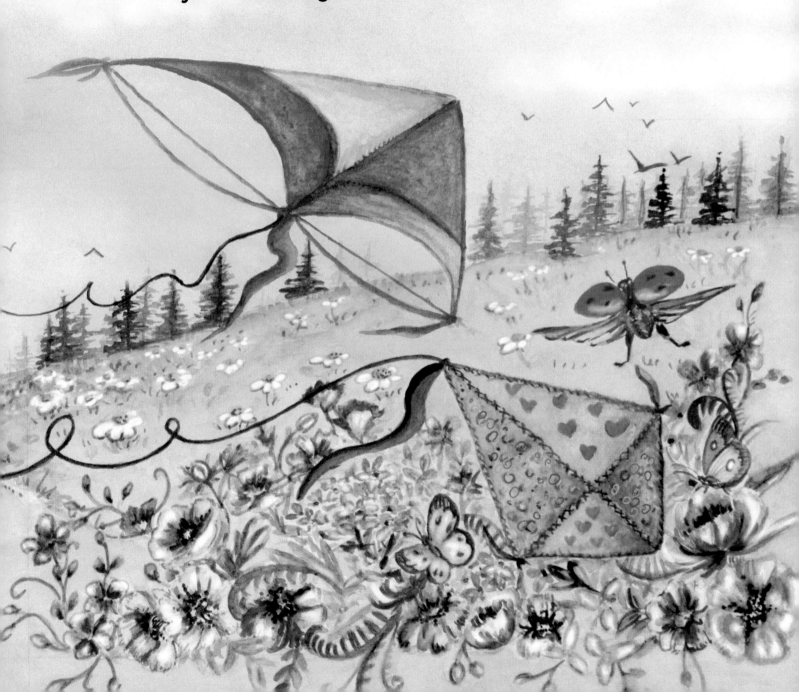

When you feel better, let's camp near the trees.
We'll swing by a stream while we feel the cool breeze.

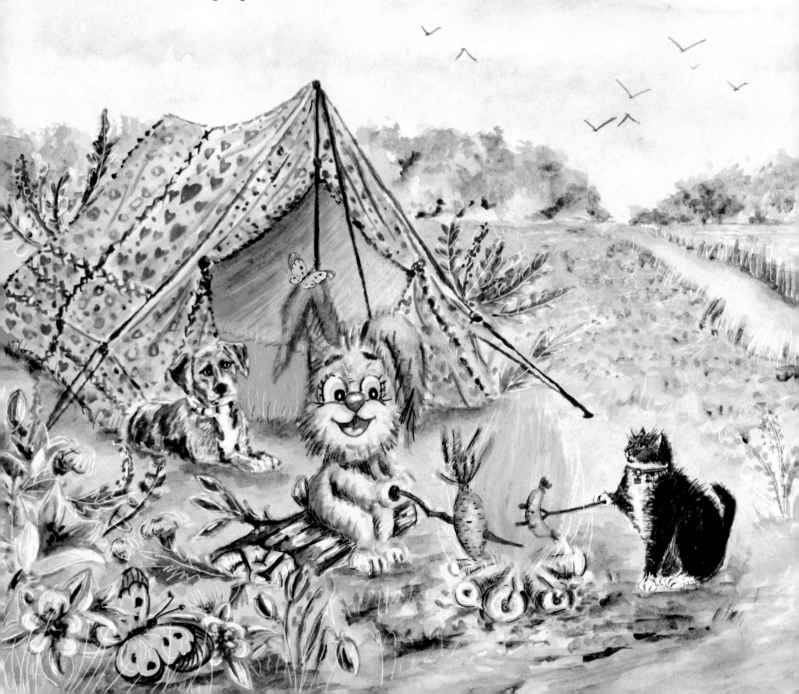

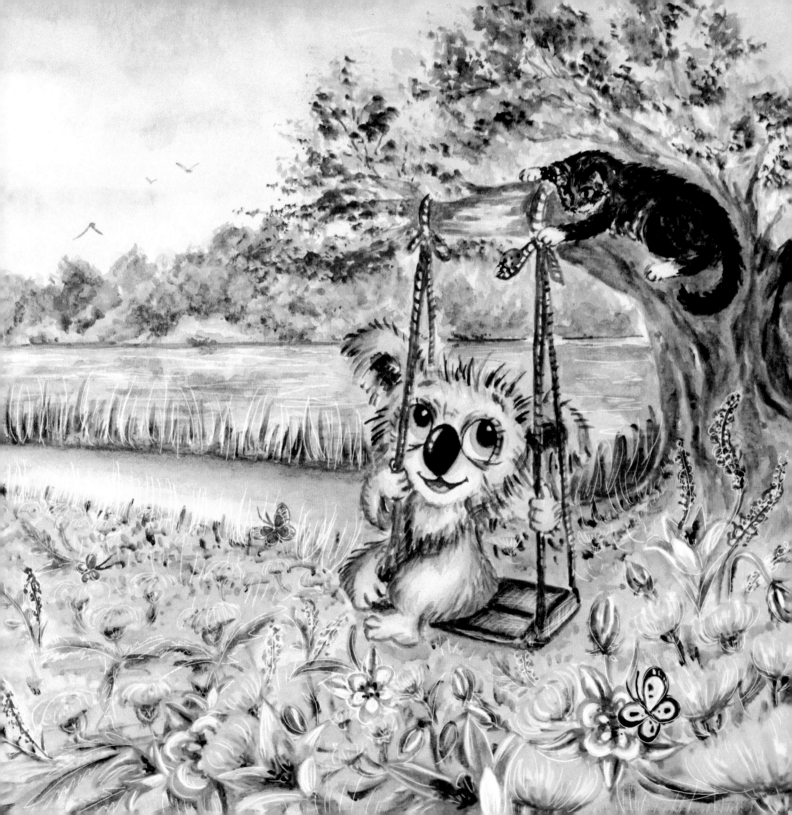

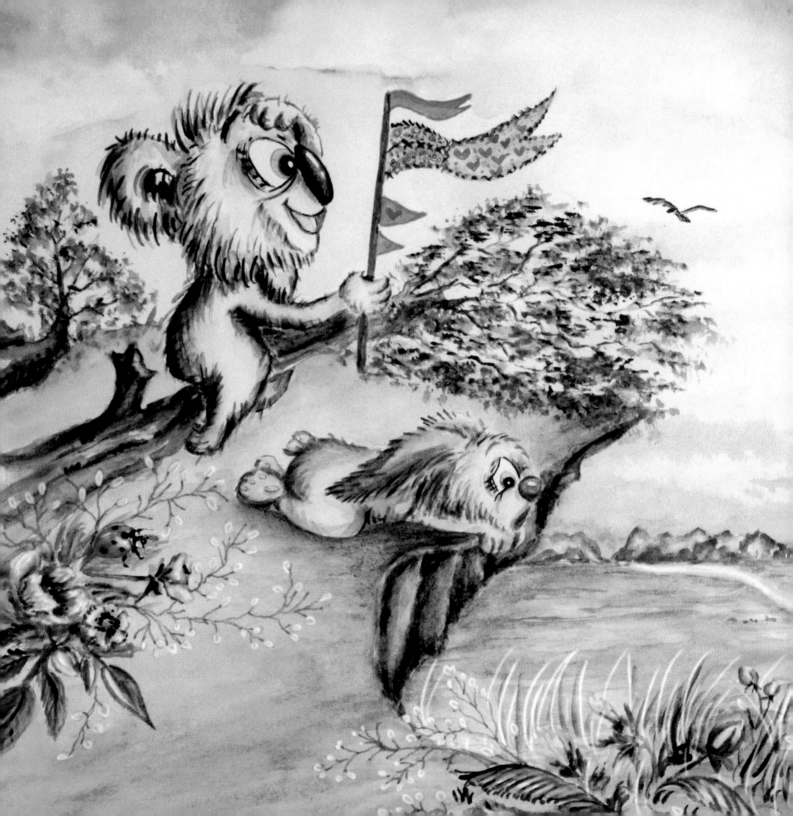

We'll follow the stream and then climb to new heights.
Let's stop and admire the beautiful sights.

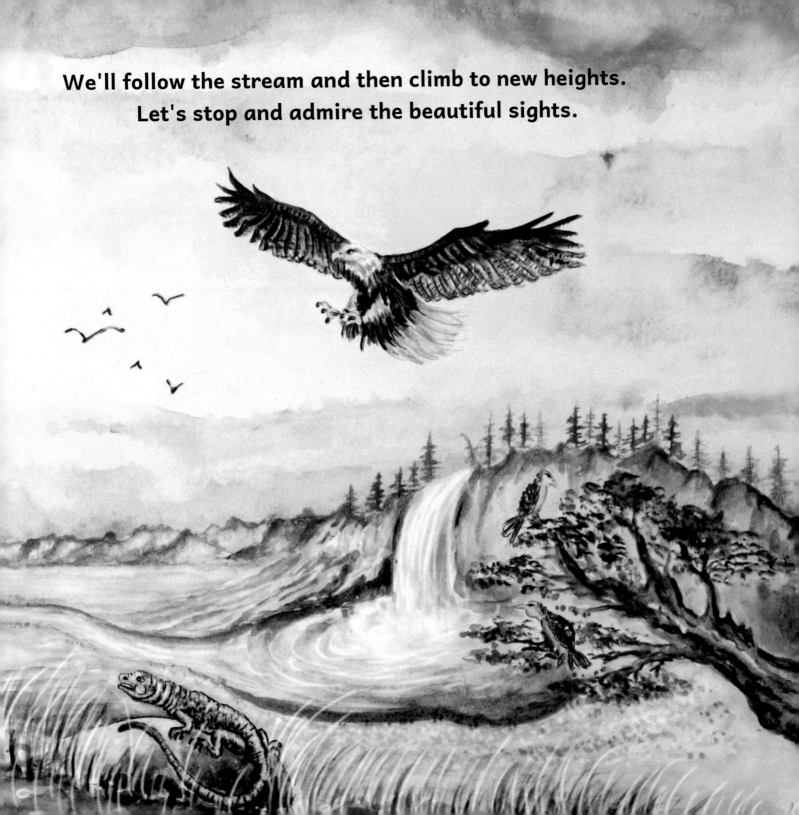

When you feel better,
let's dive in the sea.

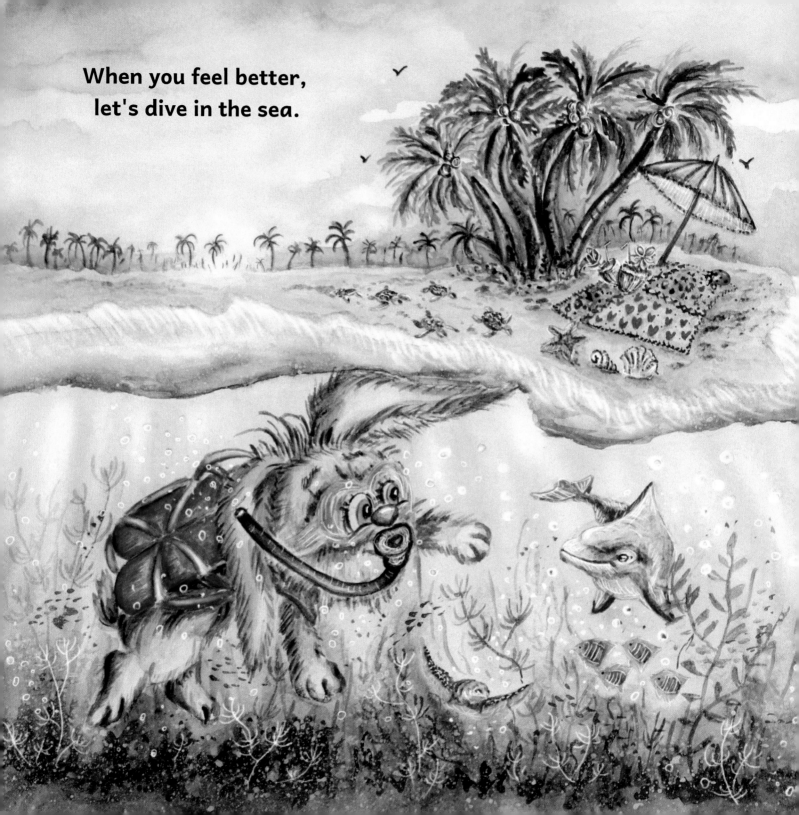

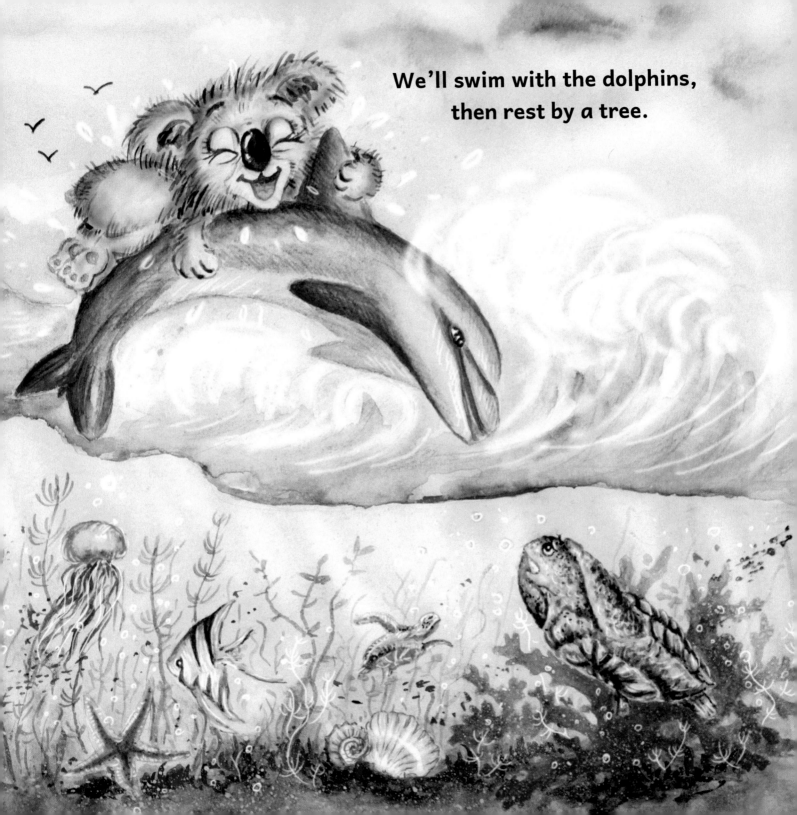

We'll swim with the dolphins,
then rest by a tree.

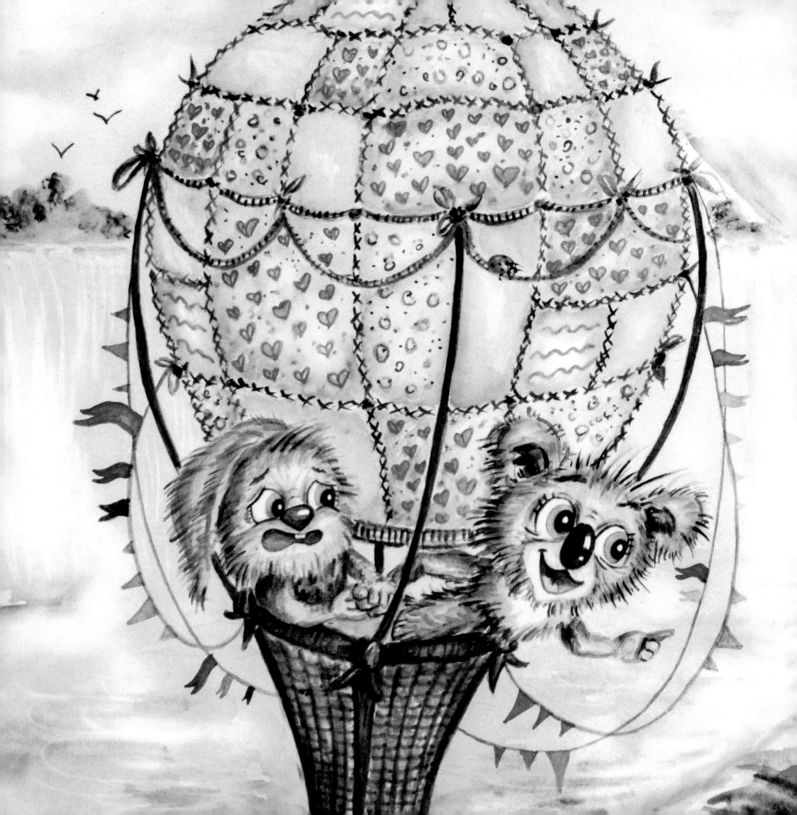

When you feel better (I hope that it's soon),
let's fly all around in our hot-air balloon.

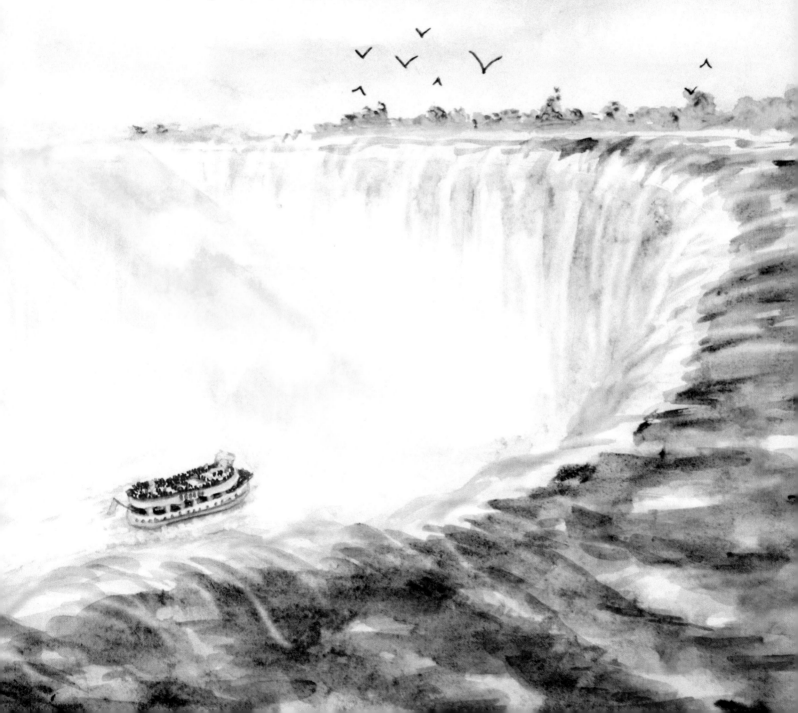

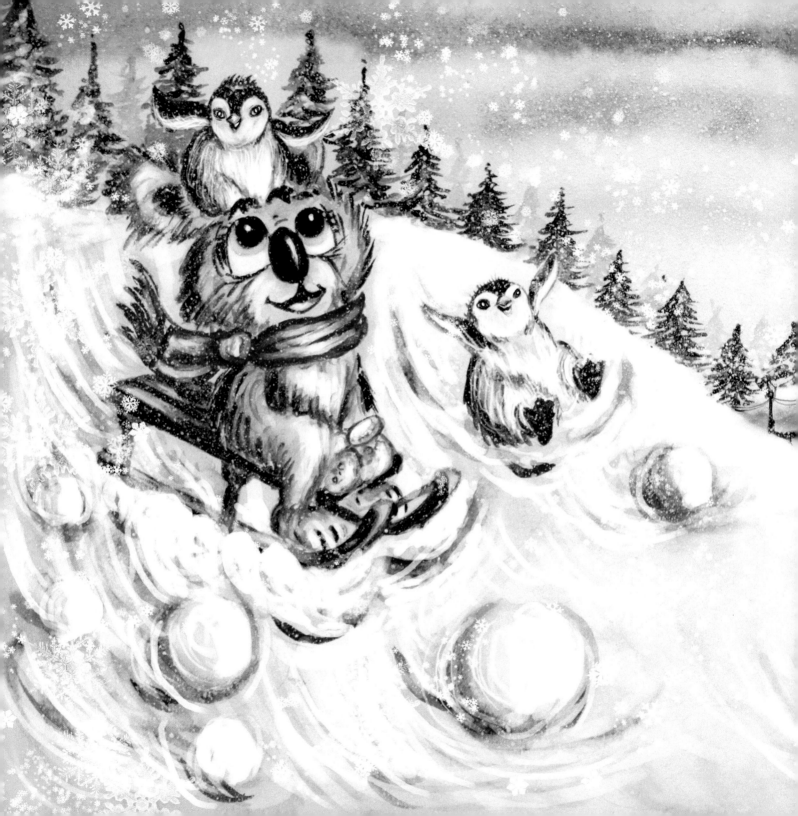

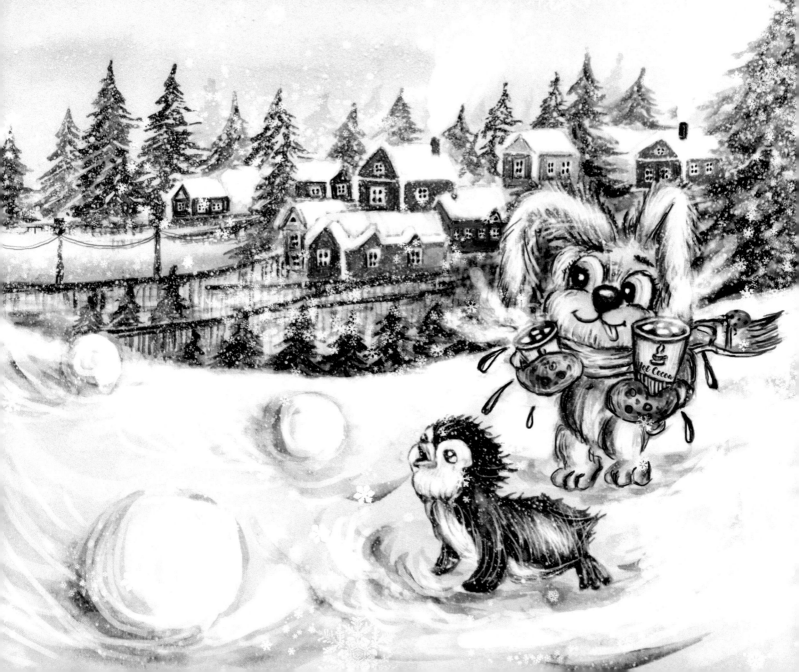

We'll head to the North; you can sled down the hill.
I'll bring the hot chocolate to help with the chill.

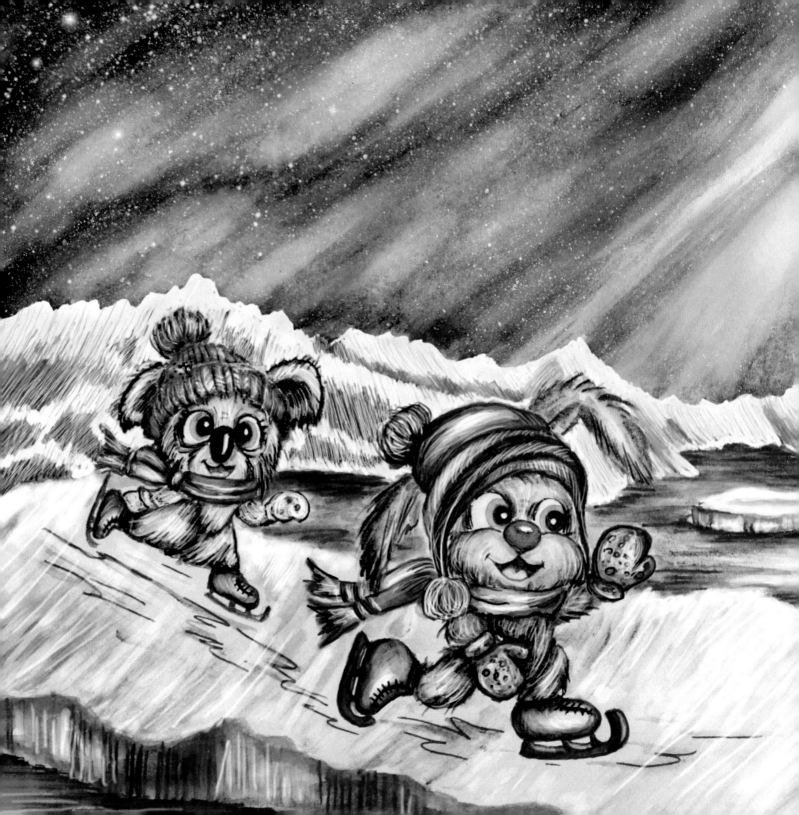

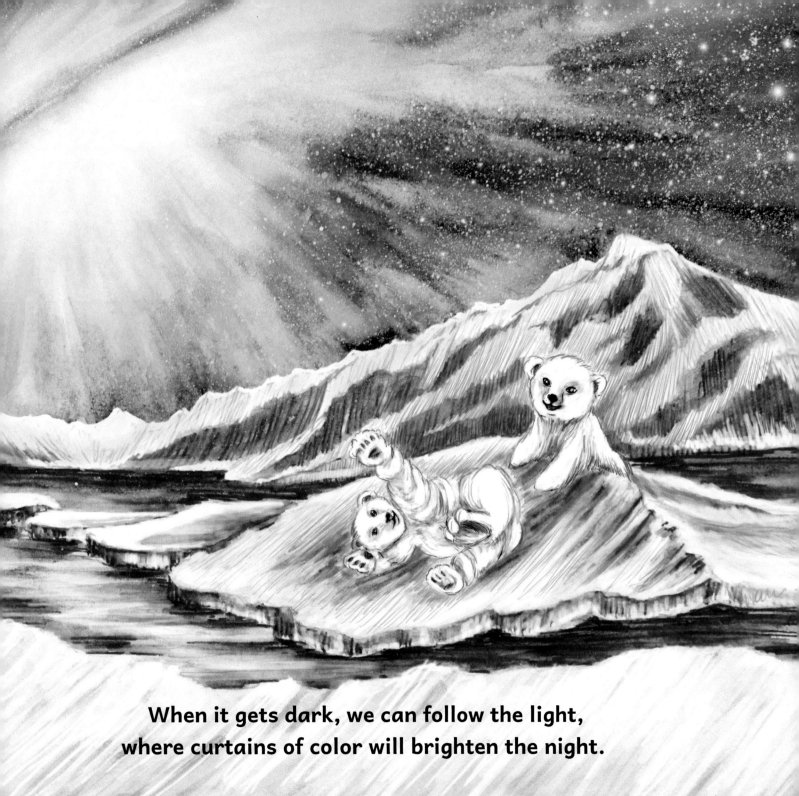

When it gets dark, we can follow the light,
where curtains of color will brighten the night.

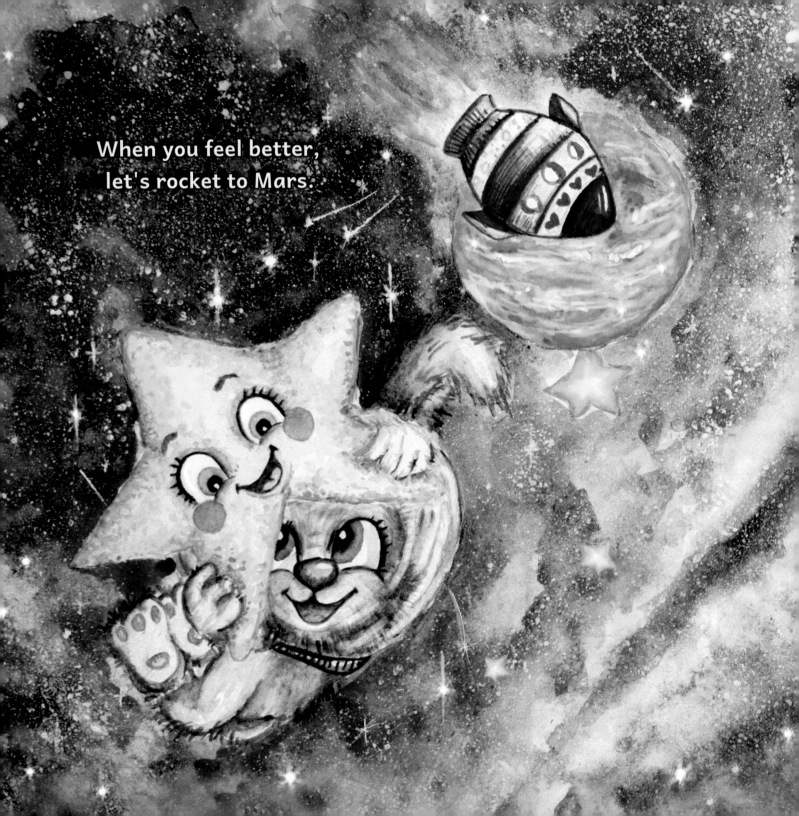

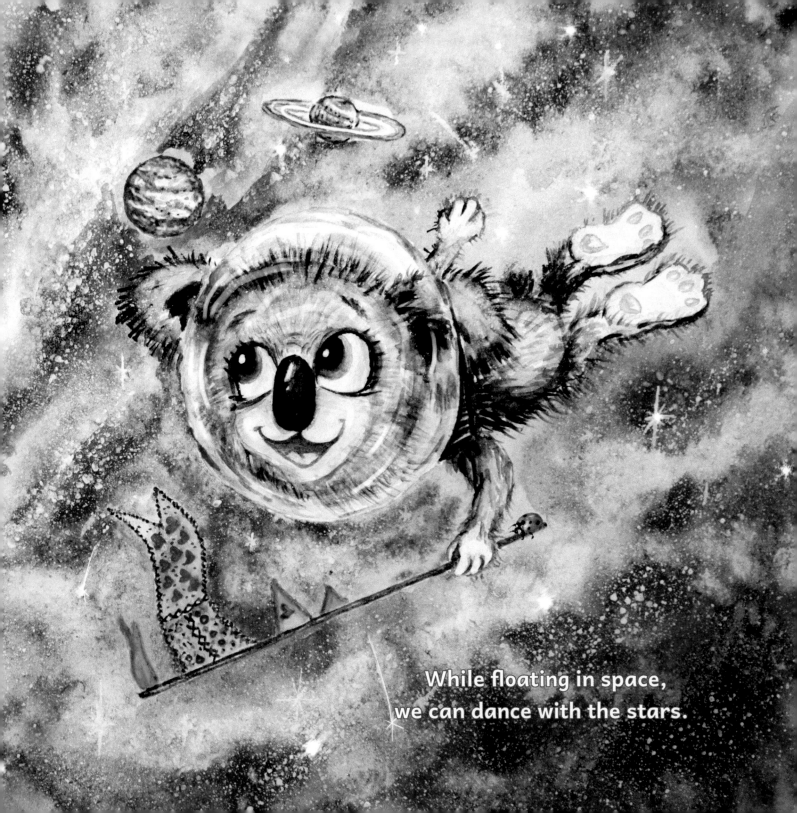

While floating in space,
we can dance with the stars.

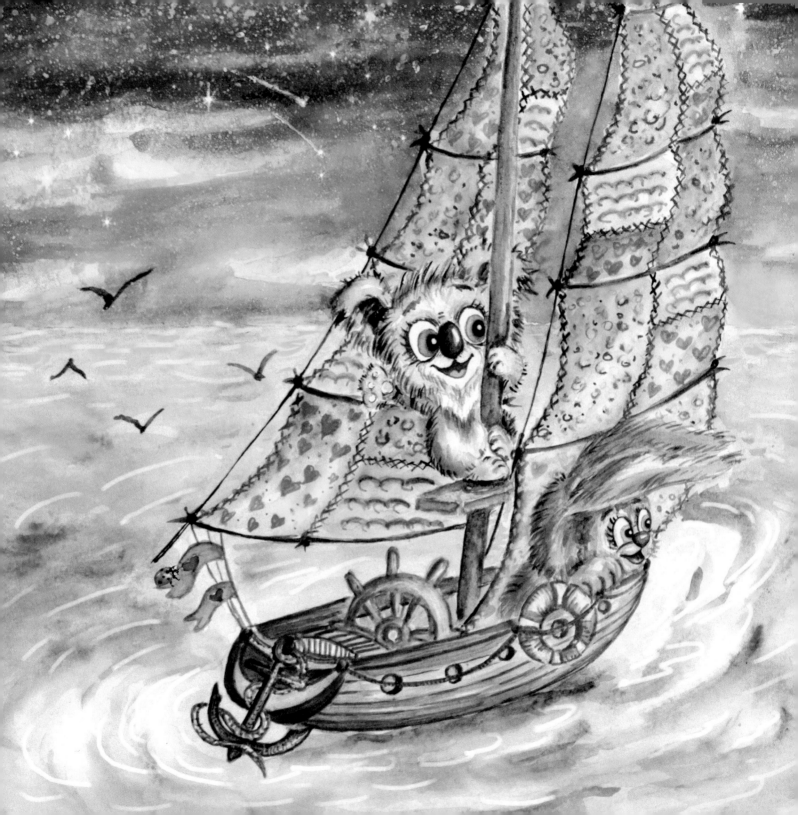

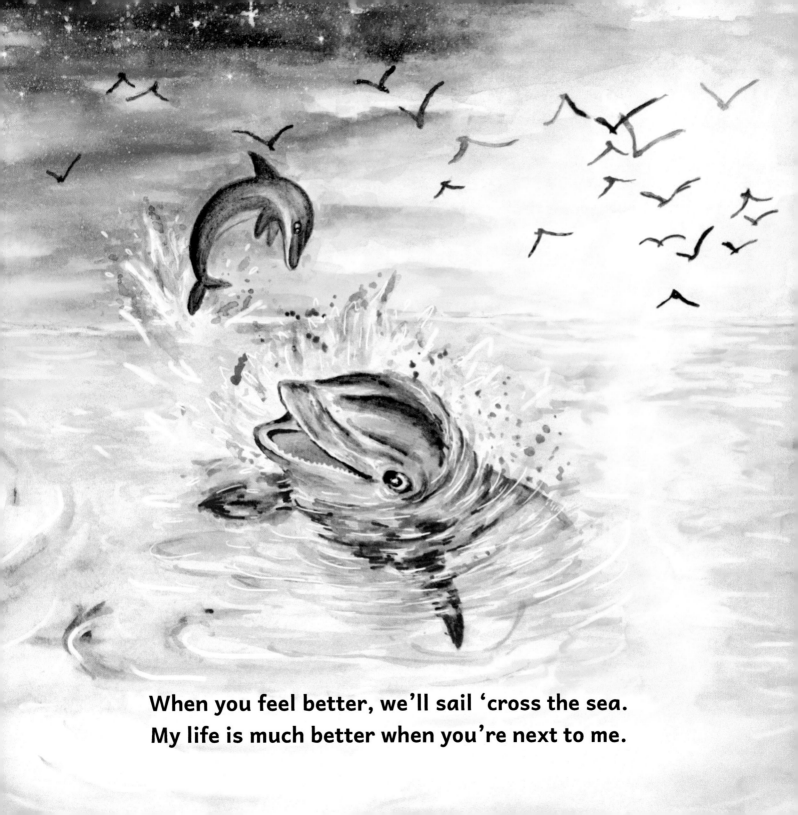

When you feel better, we'll sail 'cross the sea.
My life is much better when you're next to me.

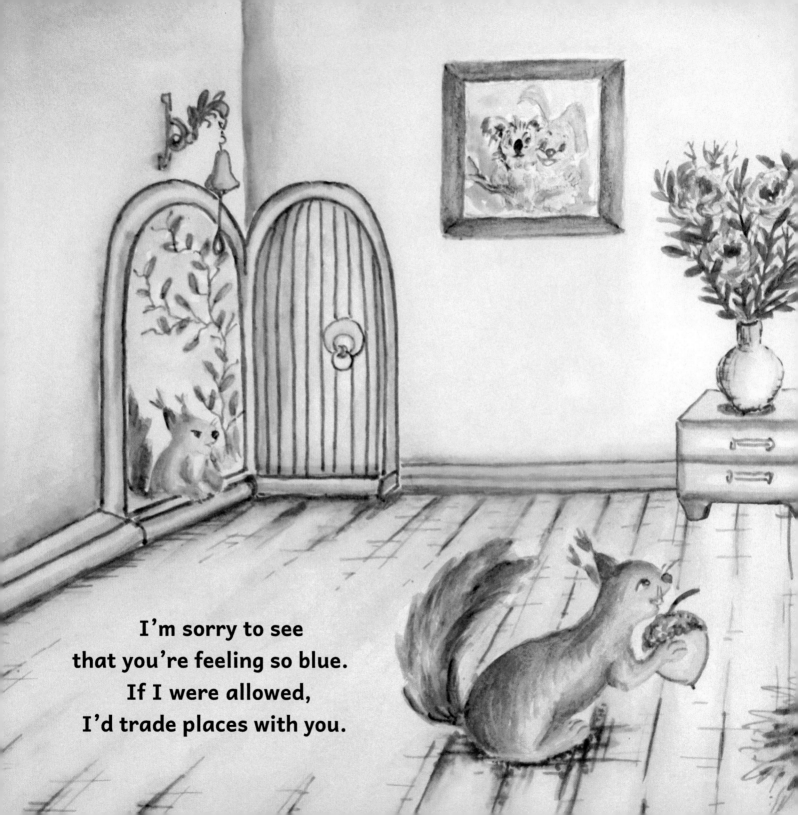

I'm sorry to see
that you're feeling so blue.
If I were allowed,
I'd trade places with you.

But since that can't happen,
I'll always be near –
to talk to you, laugh with you,
fill you with cheer.

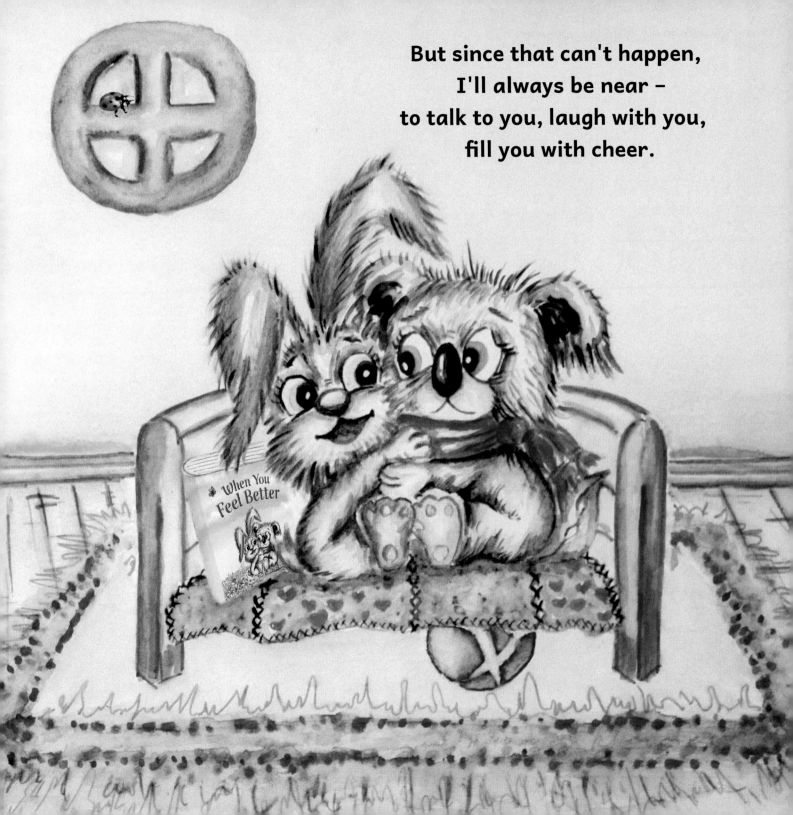

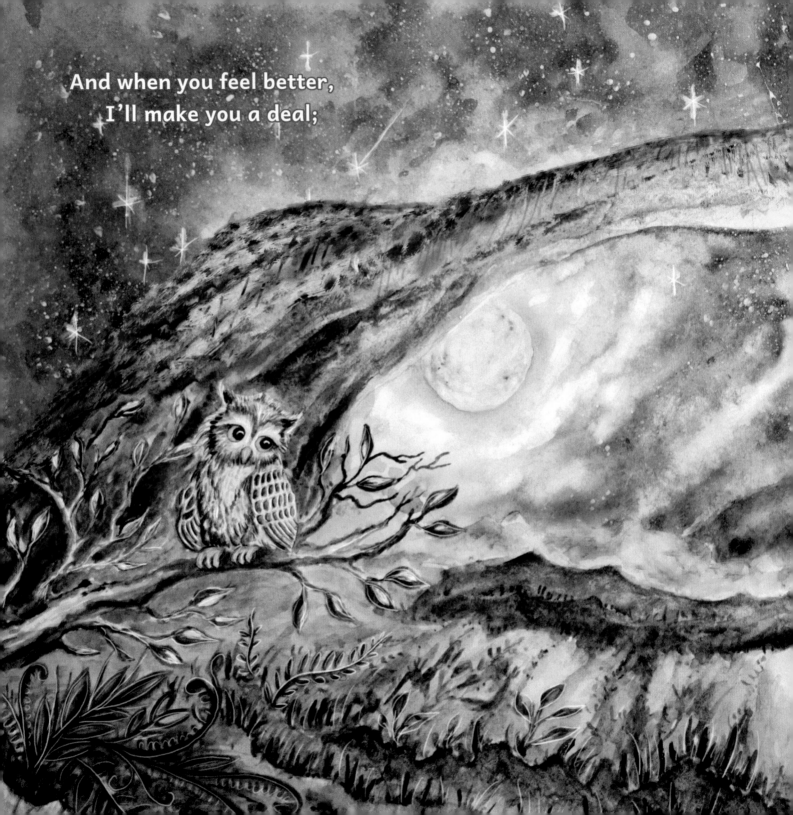

And when you feel better,
I'll make you a deal;

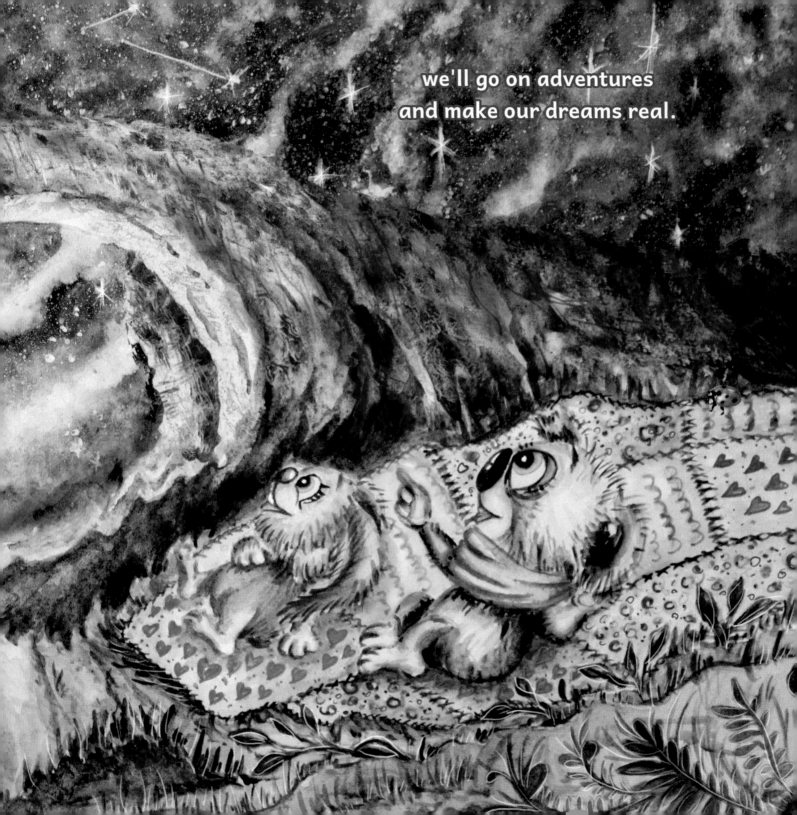

we'll go on adventures
and make our dreams real.

Dedications

Dedicated to my dear mother. I am who I am today because of you, and for that I am truly blessed.
~ Misty Black

Dedicated to children everywhere who aren't feeling well. May this book help you feel better and brighten your spirits.
~ Marina Batrak

Did you know...

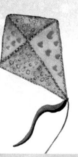

 There is a ladybug on every spread! Read the story again and see if you can find them all.

Koala's blanket is part of every adventure! Next time you read the story, see if you can find a design from the quilt on every spread.

Contest Winners

We'd like to thank everyone who participated in our contest and are proud to share that Zippy, Zoey and Chloe had the opportunity to be included in this book.

Read the story again and see if you can find them.

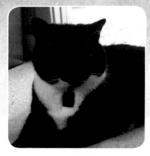

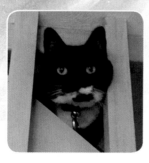

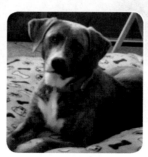

Zippy   **Zoey**   **Chloe**

About the Author

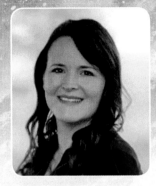

Misty Black

In addition to writing, Misty loves spending time with family and friends, playing board games, hiking, gardening (the fresh-produce part — not the weed-pulling part), and reading to her kids. If she could be anywhere, she would either be touring Europe or be in her bed reading a good book — because a good book can take you anywhere in the world.

When her mother was fighting a courageous battle with cancer, Misty never gave up hope. She wrote this book with her mother in mind saying, "Hope for better days is what gets us through the hard times. I desire that this book will bring hope to others who are fighting any type of illness or pain."

Follow at @mistyblackmedia @mistyblackmedia

To sign up for new book releases and other important information, visit berrypatchpress.com

About the Illustrator

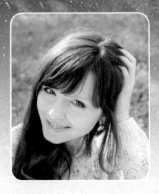

Marina Batrak

Art, painting, and creativity are Marina's life. She has loved drawing since the moment she learned how to hold a pencil. She also loves photography, playing the piano, scrapbooking, and floristry. Marina says, "The author of this book inspired me with this little story. I put a lot of work and a piece of my soul into these illustrations. I hope it brightens the spirits of everyone who reads it."

Follow at @marina_batrak

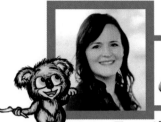
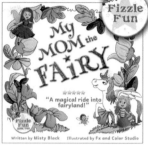
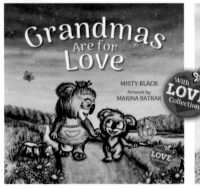
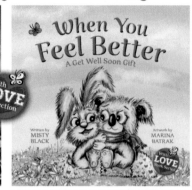
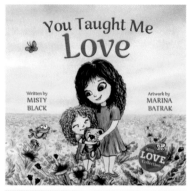
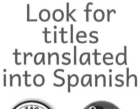

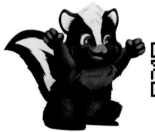

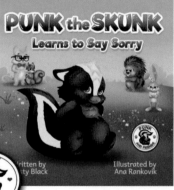
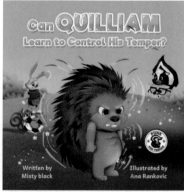
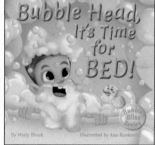
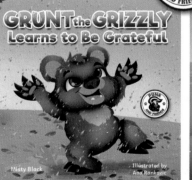
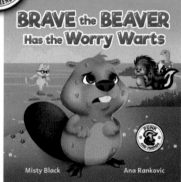
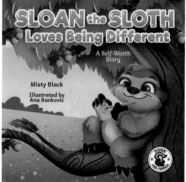

Grandma time is the BEST time!

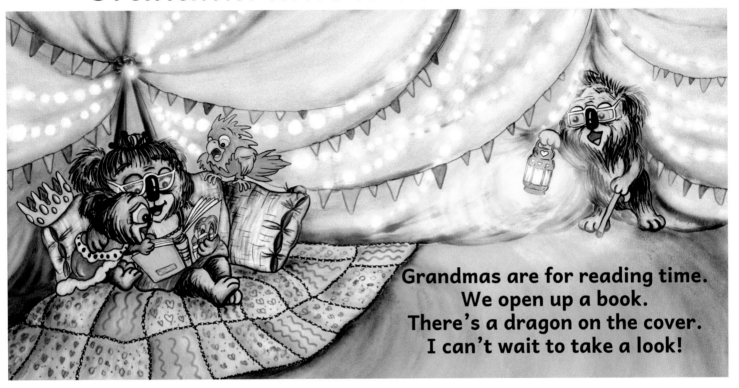

**Grandmas are for reading time.
We open up a book.
There's a dragon on the cover.
I can't wait to take a look!**

Koala and Grandma love spending time together. But how do they share their love even when they're far apart?

Read *Grandmas Are for Love* today!

Includes conversation-starter questions, a letter to a loved one, and a family tree to fill out together.

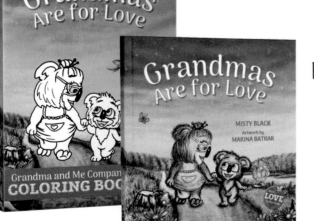

For copyright permission, school visits, and book readings/signings, email mistyblackmedia@gmail.com

Edited by Amanda Mills & Debbie Manber Kupfer
Book & Cover Design by Nicole Lavoie, Just Saying Dezigns

ISBN 978-1-951292-00-3 (paperback)
ISBN 978-1-951292-01-0 (ebook)
ISBN 978-1-951292-03-4 (Hardcover)

First Edition August 2019

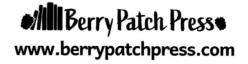

Berry Patch Press
www.berrypatchpress.com